Ketogenic Diet Cookbook

Jumpstart Your Metabolism, Burn Fat, and Lose Weight with Delicious Low-Carb Ketogenic Diet Recipes

The Wellness Foodie

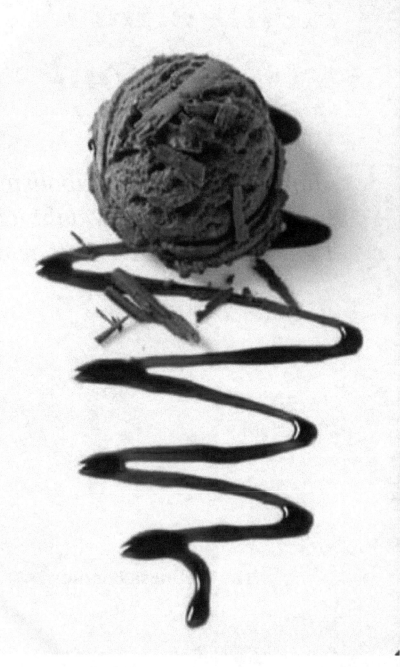

Table of Contents

Introduction

Ketogenic Diet

"Ketogenic" is a term for a low-carb diet. You can get more calories from protein and fat and less from carbohydrates by following a ketogenic diet. A keto diet is especially useful for losing excess body fat, reducing hunger, and improving type-2 diabetes or metabolic syndrome.

A keto or ketogenic diet is a low-carb, adequate protein, higher-fat diet that can help you burn fat more effectively. It has many benefits for weight loss, health, and performance.

While you eat far fewer carbohydrates on a keto diet, you maintain adequate protein consumption and may increase your intake of fat. The reduction in the carb intake puts your body in a metabolic state called ketosis, where fat, from your diet, and from your body, is burned to make energy.

People use a ketogenic diet most often to lose weight, but it can also help manage certain medical conditions, like epilepsy, heart disease, certain brain diseases, and even acne. A ketogenic diet uses more calories to change fat into energy than it does to change carbs into energy. It reduces carbs that are easy to digest, like sugar, soda, pastries, and white bread.

A keto diet can result in a calmer stomach, less gas, fewer cramps and less pain. It can increase your physical endurance by improving your access to the vast amounts of energy in your fat stores.

When you suddenly switch your body's metabolism from burning carbs (glucose) to fat and ketones, you may have some side effects as your body gets used to its new fuel. During this period, symptoms may include headache, tiredness, muscle fatigue, cramping, and heart palpitations. These side effects are short-term for most people, and there are ways to minimize or cure them.

Benefits of a Ketogenic Diet

- Weight loss and maintenance
- Reduced carbohydrate consumption plays a role in reducing your appetite
- Improvement in the quality of sleep
- Higher energy levels
- Improves emotional disposition
- Improves heart health
- Improves liver health
- Improves cognition
- Controls blood sugar and may reverse type-2 diabetes

Ketogenic Diet Risks:

- Nutrient deficiency
- Liver problems
- Kidney problems
- Constipation
- Fuzzy thinking and mood swings

Foods Allowed in the Ketogenic Diet:

- Low-carb vegetables
- Shirataki noodles
- Unsweetened tea
- Butter and cream
- Seafood
- Eggs
- Cheese
- Avocados
- Meat and poultry
- Dark chocolate and cocoa powder
- Unsweetened coffee
- Nuts and seeds
- Berries
- Olives
- Coconut oil
- Plain Greek yogurt and cottage cheese

Foods Not Allowed in the Ketogenic Diet

- Honey, syrup, or sugar in any form
- Chips and crackers
- Baked goods, including gluten-free
- Corn
- Grains
- Juices
- Rice
- Potato and sweet potato
- Starchy vegetables and high-sugar fruits
- Sweetened yogurt

10 Day Meal Plan

Days	Breakfast	Lunch	Dinner
Day 1	Scrambled eggs in butter on a bed of lettuce topped with avocado	Spinach salad with grilled salmon	Pork chop with cauliflower mash and red cabbage slaw
Day 2	Bulletproof coffee (made with butter and coconut oil), hard-boiled eggs	Tuna salad in stuffed tomatoes	Meatballs on zucchini noodles, topped with cream sauce
Day 3	Cheese and veggie omelet topped with salsa	Sashimi takeout with miso soup	Roasted chicken with asparagus and sautéed mushrooms
Day 4	Smoothie made with almond milk, greens, almond butter, and protein powder	Chicken tenders made with almond flour with greens, goat	Grilled shrimp topped with a lemon butter sauce with a side

		cheese & cucumbers	of asparagus
Day 5	Fried eggs with bacon and a side of greens	Grass-fed burger in a lettuce "bun" topped with avocado and a side salad	Baked tofu with cauliflower rice, broccoli, and peppers, topped with homemade peanut sauce
Day 6	Baked eggs in avocado cups	Poached salmon avocado rolls wrapped in seaweed (rice-free)	Grilled beef kebabs with peppers and sautéed broccolini
Day 7	Eggs scrambled with veggies, topped with salsa	Sardine salad made with mayo in half an avocado	Broiled trout with butter, sautéed bok choy
Day 8	Keto egg	Lettuce	Italian keto

	muffins	wraps with BBQ chicken	meatballs with mozzarella cheese
Day 9	Scrambled eggs in butter on a bed of lettuce topped with avocado	Keto chicken burger with jalapeno aioli	Crispy tuna burgers
Day 10	Cheese crusted omelet	Asian keto chicken stir-fry with broccoli	Tex-Mex stuffed zucchini boats

Breakfast

Breakfast Sausage and Cheese Bites

Servings: 3

Preparation Time: 20 minutes

Per Serving: 412 Calories; 34.6g Fat; 4.7g Carbs; 19.6g Protein; 0.1g Fiber

Ingredients:

- 1/2 pound breakfast sausage
- 1/2 cup almond flour
- 1/2 cup Colby cheese, shredded
- 4 tablespoons Romano cheese, freshly grated
- 1 egg

Procedure:

1. Preheat your oven to 365 degrees F.
2. Thoroughly combine all ingredients until everything is well mixed.
3. Roll the mixture into balls; place the balls on a parchment-lined baking pan sheet.
4. Bake in the preheated oven for about 15 to 17 minutes. Bon appétit!

Double Cheese and Egg Stuffed Avocados

Servings: 5

Preparation Time: 20 minutes

Per Serving: calories: 343 | fat: 30.5g | protein: 11.2g | carbs: 17.5g | net carbs: 7.4g | fiber: 10.1g

Ingredients:

- 3 avocados, halved and pitted, skin on
- ½ cup Feta cheese, crumbled
- ½ cup Cheddar cheese, grated
- 2 eggs, beaten
- Salt and black pepper, to taste
- 1 tablespoon fresh basil, chopped

Procedure:

1. Set oven to 360°F (182°C) and lay the avocado halves in an ovenproof dish.
2. In a mixing dish, mix both types of cheeses, black pepper, eggs, and salt. Split the mixture equally into the avocado halves.
3. Bake thoroughly for 15 to 17 minutes.
4. Decorate with fresh basil before serving.

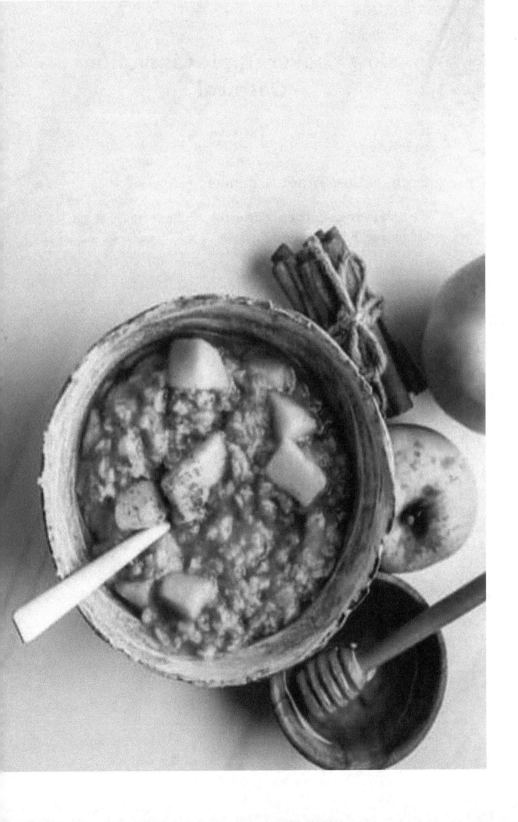

Slow Cooker Apple Cinnamon Oatmeal

Servings: 6

Preparation Time: 10 minutes

Per Serving: Cal 260, Sugar 16g, Sodium 112g, Fat 4g, Carbs 49g, Fiber 8g, Protein 8g

Ingredients:

- 3 cups plain unsweetened almond milk
- 3 cups of water
- 1 ½ cups steel-cut oats
- ⅓ cup maple syrup
- 2 tsp ground cinnamon
- A pinch of salt
- 2 large apples, shredded

Procedure:

1. In a slow cooker, mix oats, almond milk, water, maple syrup, cinnamon and salt.
2. Cover and cook for 6-8 hours on low or 3-4 on high. Stir as often as possible.

3. When fully cooked, cut and shred apples.

4. Add and mix in the slow cooker— cook for another 30 min

5. Serve with nut butter, cinnamon and shredded apple.

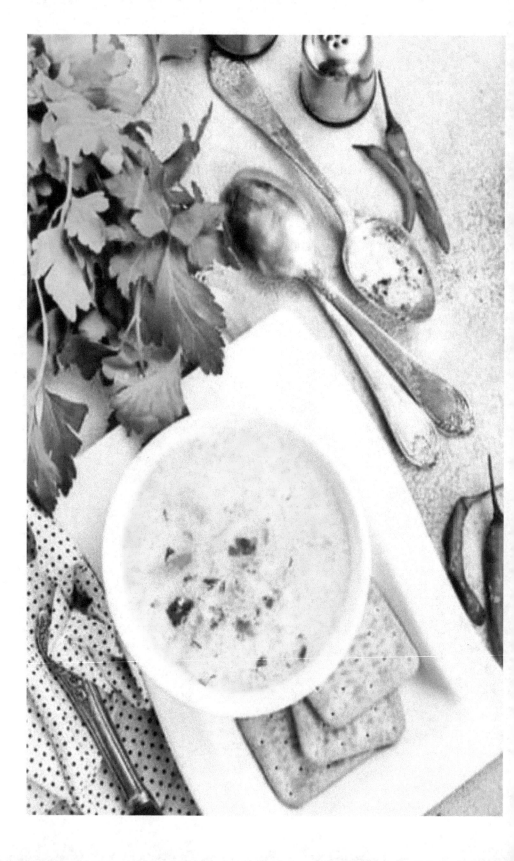

Famous Cheese Soup

Servings: 5

Preparation Time: 20 minutes

Per Serving: 439 Calories; 37g Fat; 5.7g Carbs; 19.5g Protein; 2g Fiber

Ingredients:

- 1/2 stick butter, at room temperature
- 4 tablespoons almond meal
- 2 ½ cups canned milk
- 1 chicken bouillon cube
- 2 cups Swiss cheese, shredded

Procedure:

1. In a heavy-bottomed por, melt the butter over medium-high heat.
2. Add in the almond meal, canned milk, and chicken bouillon cube,

3. Now, pour in 2 cups of warm water and let it simmer, partially covered, for 10 minutes.

4. Remove from the heat and fold in the cheese.

5. Stir to combine, cover, and let it sit in the residual heat for 8 to 10 minutes.

6. Season with salt and black pepper, and serve in individual bowls. Bon appétit!

Gruyere and Parmesan Cauliflower Burgers

Servings: 6

Preparation Time: 45 minutes

Per Serving: calories: 415 | fat: 33.7g | protein: 12.9g | carbs: 9.7g | net carbs: 7.6g | fiber: 2.1g

Ingredients:

- 1½ tablespoons olive oil
- 1 onion, chopped
- 1 garlic clove, minced
- 1 pound (454 g) cauliflower, grated
- 6 tablespoons coconut flour
- ½ cup Gruyere cheese, shredded
- 1 cup Parmesan cheese
- 2 eggs, beaten
- ½ teaspoon dried rosemary
- Sea salt and ground black pepper, to taste

Procedure:

1. Set a cast iron skillet over medium heat and warm oil.

2. Add in garlic and onion and cook until soft, about 3 minutes.

3. Stir in grated cauliflower and cook for a minute; allow cooling and set aside.

4. To the cooled cauliflower, add the rest of the ingredients; form balls from the mixture, then, press each ball to form burger patty.

5. Set oven to 400°F (205°C) and bake the burgers for 20 minutes.

6. Flip and bake for another 10 minutes or until the top becomes golden brown.

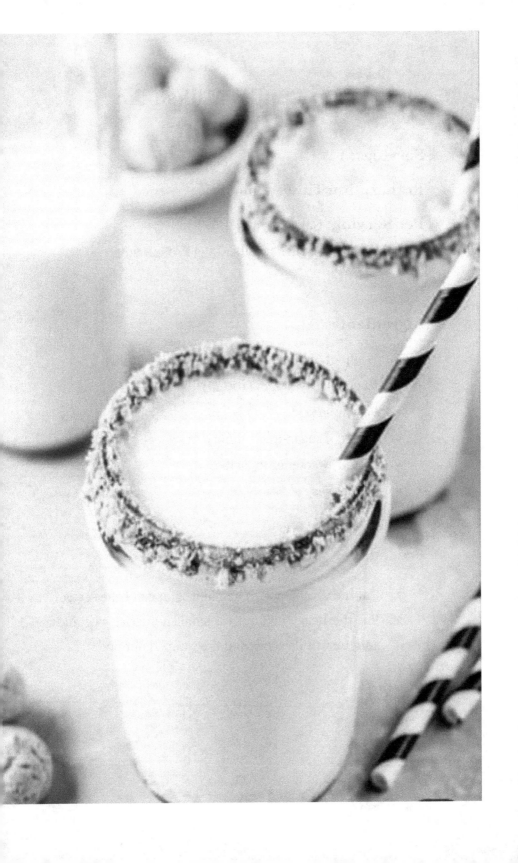

Keto Vanilla Milkshake

Servings: 1

Preparation Time: 5 minutes

Per Serving: Cal 365, Fat 38.7g, Total
Carbohydrate 3.1g Dietary Fiber 0.3g Protein 2.8g

Ingredients:

- ⅔ cup of unsweetened almond milk (150ml)
- ½ cup heavy cream (100ml)
- ½ vanilla pod
- ½ tsp of sugar-free vanilla extract
- Liquid sweetener to taste
- 5 ice cubes

Procedure:

1. Cut the vanilla pod in half and scrape out the seeds.
2. Put the heavy cream in a small non-stick pot and add the vanilla seeds and the scraped out pod.

3. Bring to a boil while continuously stirring.
4. Remove the vanilla pods from the heavy cream and pour into a container or mug.
5. Chill in refrigerator.
6. In a food processor, add the vanilla-infused heavy cream and all remaining ingredients and combine it for approx. 30 seconds.

Roquefort Kielbasa Waffles

Servings: 2

Preparation Time: 20 minutes

Per Serving: calories: 471 | fat: 40.2g | protein: 24.5g | carbs: 3.0g | net carbs: 2.8g | fiber: 0.2g

Ingredients:

- 2 tablespoons butter, melted
- Salt and black pepper, to taste
- ½ teaspoon parsley flakes
- ½ teaspoon chili pepper flakes
- 4 eggs
- ½ cup Roquefort cheese, crumbled
- 4 slices kielbasa, chopped
- 2 tablespoons fresh chives, chopped

Procedure:

1. In a mixing bowl, combine all ingredients except fresh chives.
2. Preheat waffle iron and spray with a cooking spray. Pour in the batter and close the lid.

3. Cook for 5 minutes or until golden-brown, do the same with the rest of the batter.
4. Decorate with fresh chives and serve while warm.

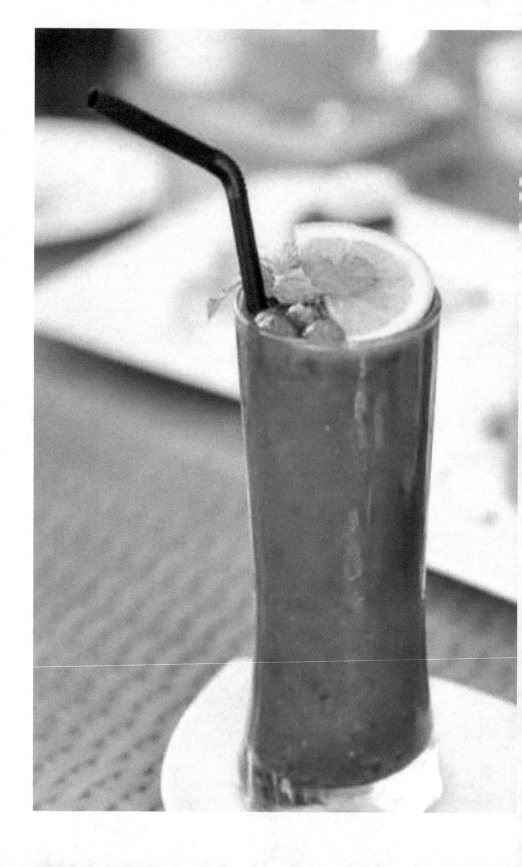

Keto Strawberry Smoothie

Servings: 2

Preparation Time: 5 minutes

Per Serving: Cal 152, Fat 13g, Carbs 5g, Fiber 1g, Protein 1g, Net carbs 4g

Ingredients:

- ¼ cup heavy whipping cream
- ¾ cup unsweetened original almond milk
- 2 tsp granulated stevia/erythritol blend (Pyure)
- 4 oz frozen strawberries
- ½ cup ice
- ½ tsp vanilla extract

Procedure:

1. Place all ingredients in blender.
2. Pulse until blended, if necessary, scraping down the sides.
3. Serve in 2 large glasses.

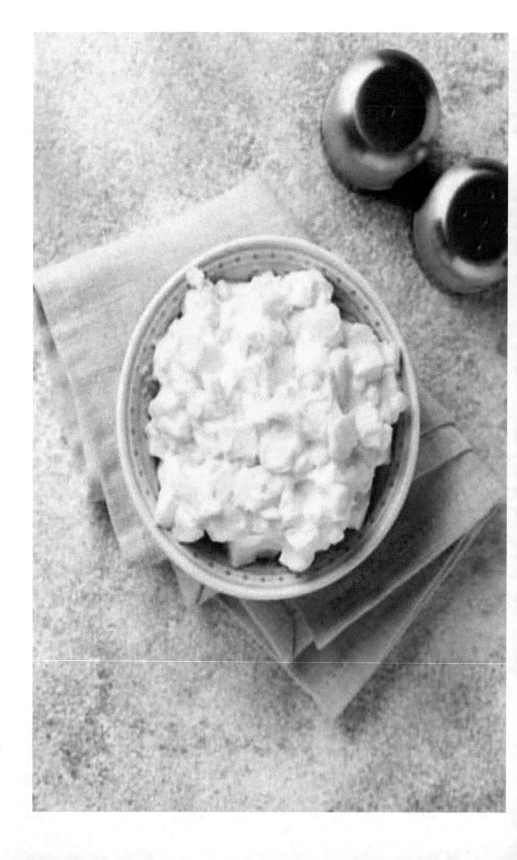

Breakfast Egg Salad

Servings: 4

Preparation Time: 15 minutes

Per Serving: 474 Calories; 37.1g Fat; 6.8g Carbs; 28g Protein; 4g Fiber

Ingredients:

- 4 eggs
- 1 Lebanese cucumber, sliced
- 4 cups lettuce, broken into pieces
- 1 avocado, pitted, peeled and sliced
- 8 ounces goat cheese, crumbled

Procedure:

1. Heat 2 tablespoons of canola oil in a frying pan over the highest heat.
2. Then, crack the eggs into the oil and fry them for 1 to 2 minutes or until the yolks are set; set aside.
3. Mix Lebanese cucumber and lettuce in a serving bowl. Place fried eggs and avocado on top.
4. Garnish with crumbled cheese and serve.

Chia Walnut Coconut Pudding

Servings: 1

Preparation Time: 10 minutes

Per Serving: calories: 335 | fat: 29.1g | protein: 15.1g | carbs: 14.5g | net carbs: 1.4g | fiber: 13.1g

Ingredients:

- ½ teaspoon vanilla extract
- ½ cup water
- 1 tablespoon chia seeds
- 2 tablespoons hemp seeds
- 1 tablespoon flax seed meal
- 2 tablespoons almond meal
- 2 tablespoons shredded coconut
- ¼ teaspoon granulated stevia
- 1 tablespoon walnuts, chopped

Procedure:

1. Put chia seeds, hemp seeds, flaxseed meal, almond meal, granulated stevia, and shredded coconut in a nonstick saucepan and pour over the water.
2. Simmer over medium heat, occasionally stirring, until creamed and thickened, for about 3-4 minutes.
3. Stir in vanilla.
4. When the pudding is ready, spoon into a serving bowl, sprinkle with walnuts and serve warm.

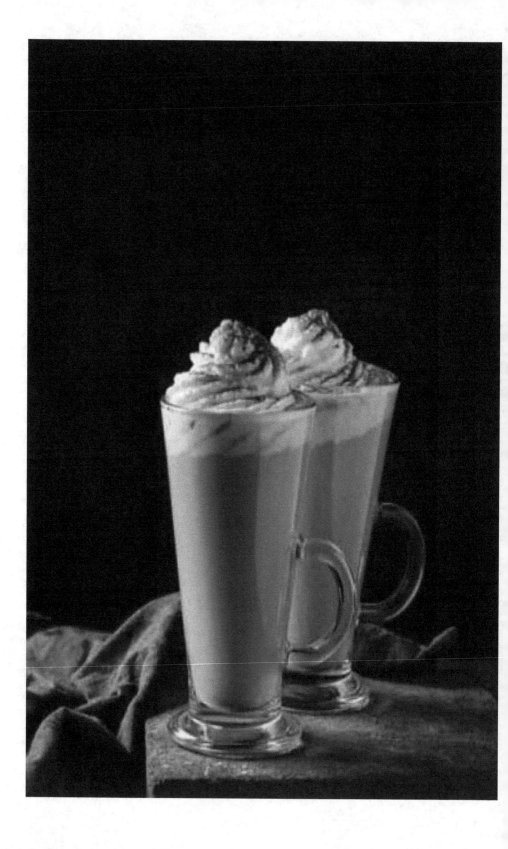

Keto Chocolate Milkshake

Servings: 2

Preparation Time: 5 minutes

Per Serving: Cal 303, Fat 31g, Saturated Fat 22g, Sodium 18mg, Potassium 491mg, Carbs 10.75g, Fiber 5.5g, Protein 3g

Ingredients:

- ½ cup Full-fat coconut milk or heavy cream
- ½ medium avocado
- 1-2 Tbsp cacao powder to taste
- ½ tsp vanilla
- 1 pinch of salt
- 2-4 Tbsp erythritol or sweetener of choice
- ½ cup ice, if desired

Procedure:

1. Place coconut milk, avocado, cacao powder, vanilla extract, salt and sweetener in blender.
2. Blend until fluffy and smooth.
3. Add ice if desired and blend until mixture is thick and creamy.
4. Do not over-mix or lose thickness and coldness. Try it instantly.

Pepperoni Ciabatta

Servings: 6

Preparation Time: 15 minutes

Per Serving: calories: 465 | fat: 33.5g | protein: 31.2g | carbs: 10.5g | net carbs: 9.2g | fiber: 1.3g

Ingredients:

- 10 ounces (283 g) cream cheese, melted
- 2½ cups Mozzarella cheese, shredded
- 4 large eggs, beaten
- 3 tablespoons Romano cheese, grated
- ½ cup pork rinds, crushed
- 2½ teaspoon baking powder
- ½ cup tomato purée
- 12 large slices pepperoni

Procedure:

1. Combine eggs, Mozzarella cheese and cream cheese.
2. Place in baking powder, pork rinds, and Romano cheese.

3. Form into 6 chiabatta shapes.

4. Set a nonstick pan over medium heat.

5. Cook each ciabatta for 2 minutes per side.

6. Sprinkle tomato purée over each one and top with pepperoni slices to serve.

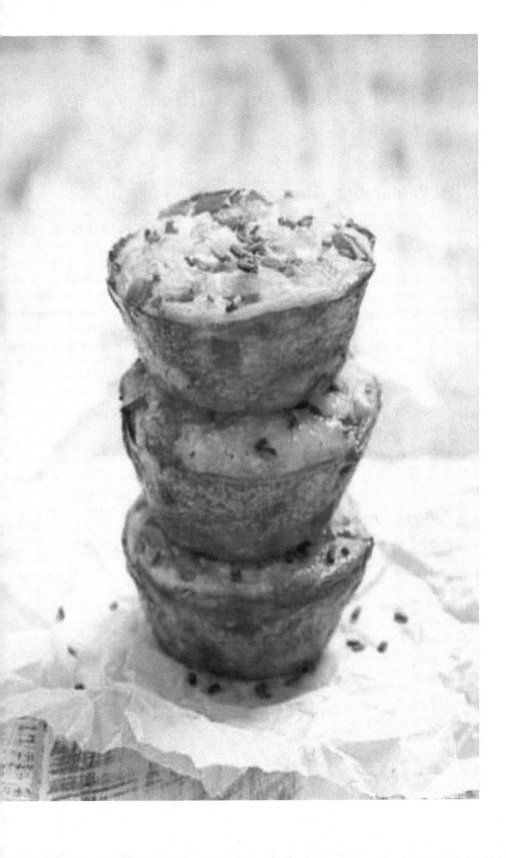

Keto Egg Muffins

Servings: 6

Preparation Time: 20 minutes

Per Serving: Fat 26g, Protein 23g, Cal 336 , Net carbs 2g

Ingredients:

- 2 scallions, finely chopped
- salt and pepper
- 6 oz shredded cheese
- 12 eggs
- 6 cooked strips sugar-free bacon, crumbled

Procedure:

1. Heat the oven to 175 F C.
2. Arrange a muffin tin with an insertable baking cups.
3. Add scallions and bacon to the base of the tin.

4. Mix the eggs with salt, and pepper. Add the cheese and stir.

5. Pour batter on top of scallions and bacon.

6. Based on the size of the muffin tin, bake for 15-20 min

Poultry

Slow Cooker Chicken Cacciatore

Servings: 4

Preparation Time: 10 minutes

Per Serving: Cal203 Fat3g Protein 29g Total Carbs 10g
Net Carbs 8g Fiber2g Sugar5g

Ingredients:

- 2 cloves garlic (minced)
- ½ large onion (diced)
- 1 large red bell pepper (diced)
- 1 (14.5 oz) can diced tomatoes (drained)
- 1 Tbsp fresh rosemary (chopped)
- 1 Tbsp fresh thyme (chopped)
- 4 medium chicken breasts
- 1 tsp sea salt
- ¼ tsp black pepper
- 1 medium bay leaf

Procedure:

1. Season the chicken fillets with salt and pepper.
2. Put the chicken in the slow cooker.

3. Mix the garlic, onion, pepper, diced tomatoes, rosemary and thyme in a medium bowl.
4. Pour the sauce evenly over the chicken.
5. Place a sheet in the middle of the oven.
6. Cover and cook 3 to 4 hours on high or 6 to 8 hours at low temperature.
7. Serve as quickly as possible.
8. If you want a thicker sauce, remove the chicken and simmer the sauce for another hour in the slow cooker.

Creamiest Chicken Salad Ever

Servings: 3

Preparation Time: 1 hour 20 minutes

Per Serving: 400 Calories; 35.1g Fat; 5.6g Carbs; 16.1g Protein; 1g Fiber

Ingredients:

- 1 chicken breast, skinless
- 1/4 mayonnaise
- 1/4 cup sour cream
- 2 tablespoons Cottage cheese, room temperature
- 1/2 avocado, peeled and cubed

Procedure:

1. Cook the chicken in a pot of salted water.
2. Remove from the heat and let the chicken sit, covered, in the hot water for 10 to 15 minutes.
3. Slice the chicken into bite-sized strips.
4. Toss with the remaining ingredients.
5. Place in the refrigerator for at least one hour. Serve well chilled. Enjoy!

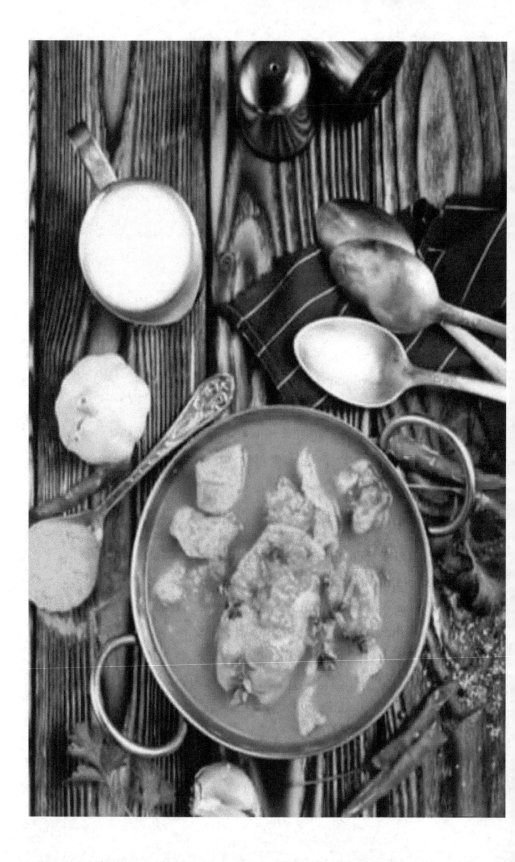

Chicken Garam Masala

Servings: 4

Preparation Time: 40 minutes

Per Serving: calories: 564 | fat: 50g | protein: 33g | carbs: 6g | net carbs: 5g | fiber: 1g

Ingredients:

- 1 pound (454 g) chicken breasts, sliced lengthwise
- 1 tablespoon butter
- 1 tablespoon olive oil
- 1 yellow bell pepper, finely chopped
- 1¼ cups heavy whipping cream
- 1 tablespoon fresh cilantro, finely chopped
- Salt and pepper, to taste
- For the Garam Masala:
- 1 teaspoon ground cumin
- 1 teaspoon ground coriander
- 1 teaspoon ground cardamom
- 1 teaspoon turmeric
- 1 teaspoon ginger

- 1 teaspoon paprika
- 1 teaspoon cayenne, ground
- 1 pinch ground nutmeg

Procedure:

1. Set your oven to 400°F (205°C). In a bowl, mix the garam masala spices.
2. Coat the chicken with half of the masala mixture.
3. Heat the olive oil and butter in a frying pan over medium-high heat, and brown the chicken for 3 to 5 minutes per side.
4. Transfer to a baking dish.
5. To the remaining masala, add heavy cream and bell pepper.
6. Season with salt and pepper and pour over chicken.
7. Bake for 20 minutes until the mixture starts to bubble.
8. Garnish with chopped cilantro to serve.

Crispy Air Fryer Chicken Wings

Servings: 4

Preparation Time: 10 minutes

Per Serving: Cal275 Fat19g Protein 22g Total Carbs 1g
Net Carbs 1g

Ingredients:

- 2 lb chicken wings
- 1 Tbsp baking powder
- 3/4 tsp Sea salt
- ¼ tsp Black pepper

Procedure:

1. Combine baking powder, sea salt, and black pepper in a large bowl.
2. Grease 2 frying ovens.
3. Place the wings on the greased trays or place enough arms in the basket to form a single layer.

4. (If you are using a pan, you may need to cook in 2 portions.)

5. Place the bucket or grill in the fryer and bake at 250 For 15 min

6. Turn the wings and turn the drawers upwards and vice versa.

7. Increase the temperature to 430 F (or your deep fryer is the highest).

8. Bake in the oven until the chicken wings are ready and crisp for about 15 to 20 min

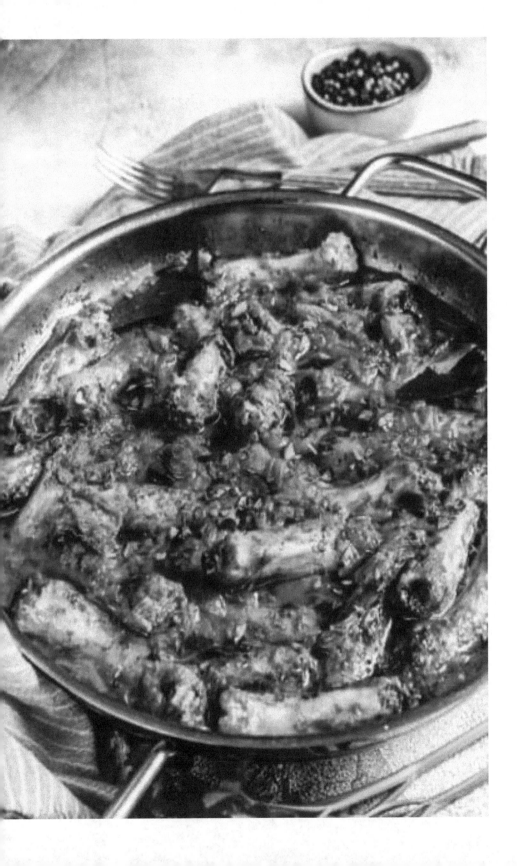

Thai Turkey Curry

Servings: 4

Preparation Time: 1 hour

Per Serving: 295 Calories; 19.5g Fat; 2.9g Carbs; 25.5g Protein; 1g Fiber

Ingredients:

- 1 pound turkey wings, boneless and chopped
- 2 cloves garlic, finely chopped
- 1 Thai red chili pepper, minced
- 1 cup unsweetened coconut milk, preferably homemade
- 1 cup turkey consommé

Procedure:

1. In a saucepan, warm 2 teaspoons of sesame oil.
2. Once hot, brown turkey about 8 minutes or until it is golden brown.

3. Add in the garlic and Thai chili pepper and continue to cook for a minute or so.
4. Add coconut milk and consommé. Season with salt and black pepper to taste.
5. Continue to cook for 40 to 45 minutes over medium heat. Serve warm and enjoy!

Lemony Chicken Wings

Servings: 4

Preparation Time: 25 minutes

Per Serving: calories: 365 | fat: 25g | protein: 21g | carbs: 4g | net carbs: 4g | fiber: 0g

Ingredients:

- A pinch of garlic powder
- 1 teaspoon lemon zest
- 1 tablespoon lemon juice
- ½ teaspoon ground cilantro
- 1 tablespoon fish sauce
- 1 tablespoon butter
- ¼ teaspoon xanthan gum
- 1 tablespoon Swerve sweetener
- 20 chicken wings
- Salt and black pepper, to taste

Procedure:

1. Combine lemon juice and zest, fish sauce, cilantro, sweetener, and garlic powder in a saucepan.
2. Bring to a boil, cover, lower the heat, and let simmer for 10 minutes.
3. Stir in the butter and xanthan gum.
4. Set aside and season the wings with some salt and pepper.
5. Preheat the grill and cook for 5 minutes per side.
6. Serve topped with the sauce.

Baked Teriyaki Turkey

Servings: 2

Preparation Time: 15 minutes

Per Serving: 410 Calories; 27.1g Fat; 6.6g Carbs; 36.5g Protein; 1g Fiber

Ingredients:

- 3/4 pound lean ground turkey
- 1 brown onion, chopped
- 1 red bell pepper, deveined and chopped
- 1 serrano pepper, deveined and chopped
- 1/4 cup keto teriyaki sauce

Procedure:

1. Cook the ground turkey in the preheated pan over medium-high heat; cook for about 5 minutes until no longer pink.
2. Now, sauté the onion and peppers for 3 minutes more.

3. Add in teriyaki sauce and bring the mixture to a boil.

4. Immediately remove from the heat; add in the cooked ground turkey and sautéed mixture.

5. Serve warm and enjoy!

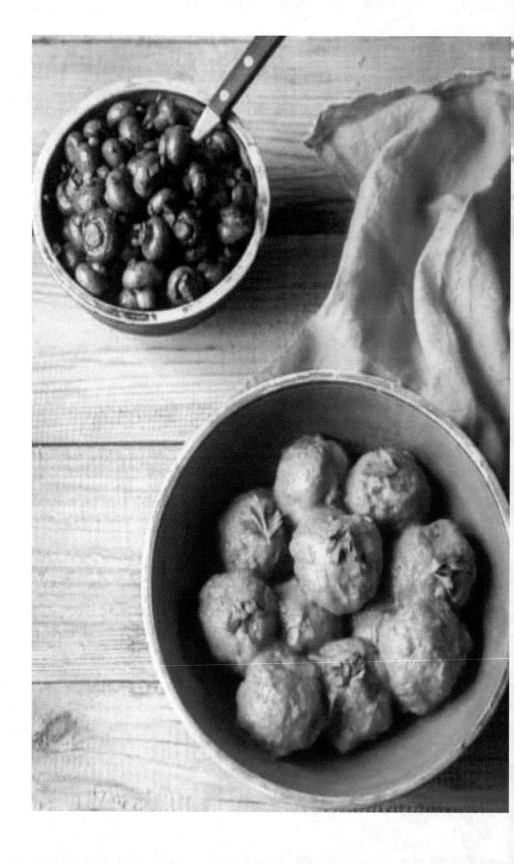

Basil Turkey Meatballs

Servings: 4

Preparation Time: 15 minutes

Per Serving: calories: 310 | fat: 26g | protein: 22g | carbs: 3g | net carbs: 2g | fiber: 1g

Ingredients:

- 1 pound (454 g) ground turkey
- 1 tablespoon chopped sun-dried tomatoes
- 1 tablespoon chopped basil
- ½ teaspoon garlic powder
- 1 egg
- ½ teaspoon salt
- ¼ cup almond flour
- 1 tablespoon olive oil
- ½ cup shredded mozzarella cheese
- ¼ teaspoon pepper

Procedure:

1. Place everything, except the oil in a bowl.
2. Mix with your hands until combined.
3. Form into 16 balls. Heat the olive oil in a skillet over medium heat.
4. Cook the meatballs for 4-5 minutes per each side.
5. Serve immediately.

Greek Chicken Bowls

Servings: 4

Preparation Time: 20 minutes

Per Serving: Cal287 Fat15g Protein 28g Total Carbs 7g Net Carbs 6g Fiber 1g Sugar 4g Cal287

Ingredients:

- 1 lb chicken breast
- 1 ½ tsp Sea salt
- 3 Tbsp Olive oil
- 1 Tbsp Balsamic vinegar (optional)
- ½ tsp Black pepper (divided)
- 2 ½ cups Zucchini (thinly sliced into, ¼ inch thick)
- ½ lb Grape tomatoes
- ½ large onion
- ¼ cup Feta cheese
- ½ Tbsp dried dill
- ½ Tbsp Dried parsley
- 1 tsp dried oregano
- 1 tsp Garlic powder

Procedure:

1. Preheat the oven to 400° F. Grease a large baking sheet.
2. Fill a large bowl with water.
3. Add salt and stir to dissolve. Add the chicken and set aside for 10 to 20 min to brine.
4. Chop zucchini, grape tomatoes, and onions.
5. Stir the dried dill, parsley, oregano, garlic powder, salt and pepper in a small bowl.
6. Stick together but not touching when the chicken is cooked, brin, pat dry, and put in 1 region of the baking sheet.
7. Rub a spoonful of olive oil into both sides of the chicken.
8. Season with half the herb mixture.
9. Toss the chopped vegetables and 2 Tbsp olive oil in a large bowl.
10. Add the remaining herb mixture. Toss well to mix.
11. Set the veggies on the baking sheet in a single layer.
12. Roast in the oven for about 20 min
13. Sprinkle with feta cheese (optional)

Roast Herbs Stiffed Chicken

Servings: 8

Preparation Time: 1 hours

Per Serving: calories: 432 | fat: 32g | protein: 30g | carbs: 10g | net carbs: 5g | fiber: 5g

Ingredients:

- 5 pounds (2.3 kg) whole chicken
- 1 bunch oregano
- 1 bunch thyme
- 1 tablespoon marjoram
- 1 tablespoon parsley
- 1 tablespoon olive oil
- 2 pounds (907 g) Brussels sprouts
- 1 lemon
- 1 tablespoon butter

Procedure:

1. Preheat your oven to 450°F (235°C).
2. Stuff the chicken with oregano, thyme, and lemon.

3. Roast for 15 minutes.

4. Reduce the heat to 325°F (163°C) and cook for 40 minutes.

5. Spread the butter over the chicken, and sprinkle parsley and marjoram.

6. Add the brussels sprouts. Return to the oven and bake for 40 more minutes.

7. Let sit for 10 minutes before carving.

Chicken Escarole Soup

Servings: 4

Preparation Time: 15 minutes

Per Serving: Cal 360 Net Carbs 19g Fat 18g Protein 30g

Ingredients:

- 1 (14 ½-oz) can Italian-style stewed tomatoes, undrained and chopped
- 1 (14-oz) can chicken broth
- 1 cup chopped cooked chicken breast
- 2 cups coarsely chopped escarole (about 1 small head)
- 2 tsp extra-virgin olive oil

Procedure:

1. Combine tomatoes and food in a large saucepan.
2. Cover and bring to a boil over high heat.
3. Reduce heat to low; simmer 5 min
4. Add chicken, escarole, and oil; cook 5 min

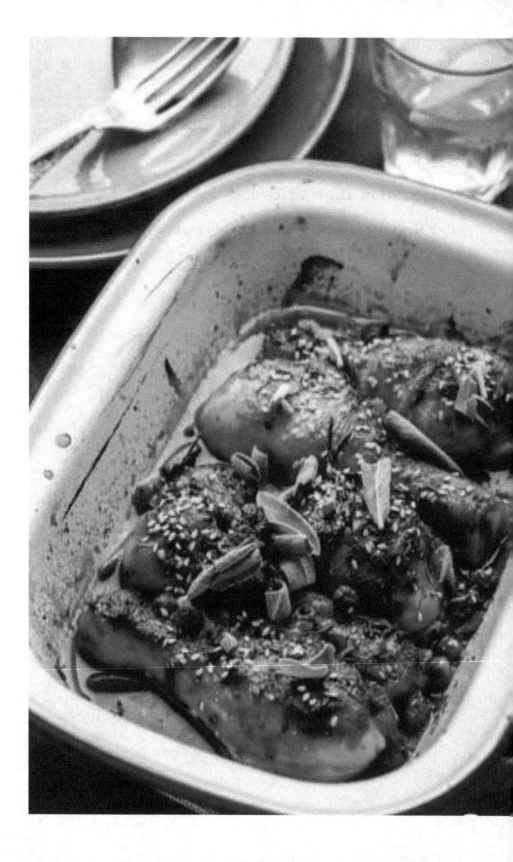

Mediterranean Herbed Chicken

Servings: 5

Preparation Time: 20 minutes

Per Serving: 370 Calories; 16g Fat; 0.9g Carbs; 51g Protein; 0.2g Fiber

Ingredients:

- 2 tablespoons butter, softened at room temperature
- 5 chicken legs, skinless
- 2 scallions, chopped
- 1 tablespoon Mediterranean spice mix
- 1 cup vegetable broth

Procedure:

1. In a saucepan, melt 1 tablespoon of butter over a medium-high flame.
2. Now, brown the chicken legs for about 10 minutes, turning them periodically.

3. Add in the remaining tablespoon of butter, scallions, Mediterranean spice mix, and broth.

4. When your mixture reaches boiling, reduce the temperature to a simmer.

5. Continue to simmer for 10 to 11 minutes until cooked through.

6. Taste and adjust the seasoning. Bon appétit!

Pesto Turkey with Zucchini Spaghetti

Servings: 6

Preparation Time: 45 minutes

Per Serving: calories: 273 | fat: 16g | protein: 19g | carbs: 7g | net carbs: 4g | fiber: 3g

Ingredients:

- 2 cups sliced mushrooms
- 1 teaspoon olive oil
- 1 pound (454 g) ground turkey
- 1 tablespoon pesto sauce
- 1 cup diced onion
- 2 cups broccoli florets
- 6 cups zucchini, spiralized

Procedure:

1. Heat the oil in a skillet.
2. Add zucchini and cook for 2-3 minutes, stirring continuously; set aside.
3. Add turkey to the skillet and cook until browned, about 7-8 minutes. Transfer to a plate.

4. Add onion and cook until translucent, about 3 minutes.
5. Add broccoli and mushrooms, and cook for 7 more minutes. Return the turkey to the skillet.
6. Stir in the pesto sauce.
7. Cover the pan, lower the heat, and simmer for 15 minutes.
8. Stir in zucchini pasta and serve immediately.

Meat

Air Fryer Buffalo Cauliflower Wings

Servings: 4

Preparation Time: 5 minutes

Per Serving: Cal 48 Carbs 1 g Fat 4 g Sodium 265 mg
Potassium 94 mg Vitamin A: 15 IU Vitamin C: 20.2 mg
Calcium: 10 mg Iron: 0.2 mg

Ingredients:

- 3-4 Tbsp hot sauce
- 1 Tbsp almond flour
- 1 Tbsp avocado oil
- Salt to taste
- 1 medium-sized cauliflower, washed and thoroughly dried

Procedure:

1. Preheat the fryer to 400° F.
2. Mix hot sauce, almond flour, avocado oil, and salt in a large bowl.
3. Add the cauliflower and mix until covered.

4. Put half of the cauliflower in the fryer and cook for 12 to 15 min (or until it is crisp on the edges with a small cock or reaches the desired level).

5. Be sure to open the fryer and shake the fry basket halfway to rotate the cauliflower.

6. Delete and book.

7. Add the second portion, but cook 2 to 3 min less.

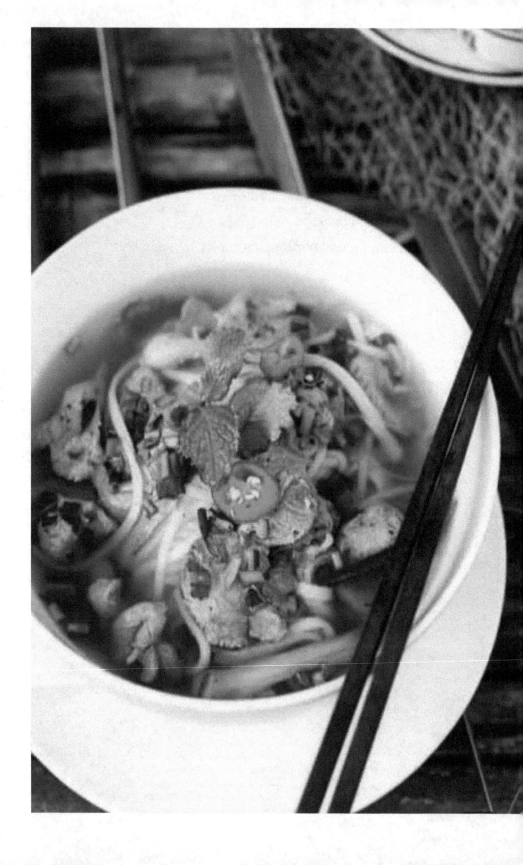

Country Style Beef Soup

Servings: 4

Preparation Time: 45 minutes

Per Serving: 181 Calories; 8.6g Fat; 2.1g Carbs; 23.2g Protein; 0.5g Fiber

Ingredients:

- 3/4 pound chuck, cut into bite-sized cubes
- 1/2 tablespoon lard, at room temperature
- 4 cups beef bone broth
- 1 celery rib, chopped
- 1/2 cup scallions, chopped

Procedure:

1. Melt the lard in a soup pot over a medium-high heat.
2. Now, sear the beef for 5 to 6 minutes, stirring periodically to ensure even cooking; reserve.
3. After that, sauté the celery and scallions in the pan drippings for about 3 minutes or until they've softened.

4. Deglaze the pan with the beef broth.

5. Return the reserved beef to the soup pot, bringing to a rolling boil.

6. Reduce the heat to medium-low and let it cook approximately 30 minutes.

7. Divide between individual bowls. Bon appétit!

Sirloin Steak with Sauce Diane

Servings: 6

Preparation Time: 30 minutes

Per Serving: calories: 436 | fat: 34g | protein: 25g | carbs: 6g | net carbs: 5g | fiber: 1g

Ingredients:

Sirloin Steak:

- 1½ pounds (680 g) sirloin steak
- Salt and black pepper, to taste
- 1 teaspoon olive oil

Sauce Diane:

- 1 tablespoon olive oil
- 1 clove garlic, minced
- 1 cup sliced porcini mushrooms
- 1 small onion, finely diced
- 2 tablespoons butter
- 1 tablespoon Dijon mustard

- 2 tablespoons Worcestershire sauce
- ¼ cup whiskey
- 2 cups heavy whipping cream
- Salt and black pepper, to taste

Procedure:

1. Put a grill pan over high heat and as it heats, brush the steak with oil, sprinkle with salt and pepper, and rub the seasoning into the meat with your hands.
2. Cook the steak in the pan for 4 minutes on each side for medium rare and transfer to a chopping board to rest for 4 minutes before slicing.
3. Reserve the juice.
4. Heat the oil in a frying pan over medium heat and sauté the onion for 3 minutes.
5. Add the butter, garlic, and mushrooms, and cook for 2 minutes.
6. Add the Worcestershire sauce, the reserved juice, and mustard.
7. Stir and cook for 1 minute.

8. Pour in the whiskey and cook further 1 minute until the sauce reduces by half. Swirl the pan and add the cream.
9. Let it simmer to thicken for about 3 minutes.
10. Adjust the taste with salt and pepper.
11. Spoon the sauce over the steaks slices and serve with celeriac mash.

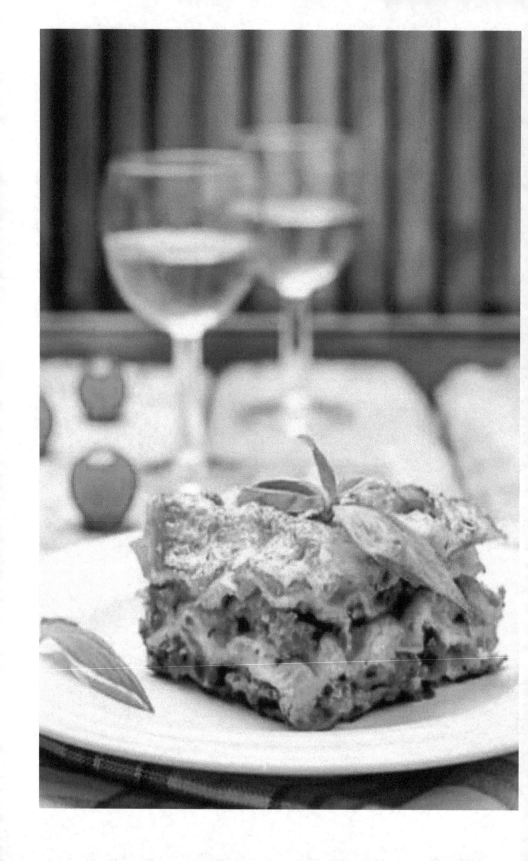

Keto Lasagna

Servings: 6

Preparation Time: 15 minutes

Per Serving: Cal 514.1 Fat 28.5g Carbs 4.9 Fiber .3g
Protein 21.1g

Ingredients:

- 1 lb ground beef
- ½ lb Italian sausage
- ¼ cup chopped white onion
- 1 ½ cups marinara sauce
- 3/4 tsp garlic powder, divided
- 1 tsp oregano, divided
- ½ cup ricotta cheese
- 1 cup grated mozzarella, divided
- 2/3 cup parmesan, divided
- Chopped parsley for garnish (optional)

Procedure:

1. Preheat the oven to 400° F.
2. In a 12-inch cast-iron skillet (or similar oven-proof equivalent), brown the ground meat and the ground

sausage over medium heat on the stove until it isn't pink (about 15 min).

3. Drain off excess fat and heat again.

4. Put the onions in the pan and fry it with meat until it starts to soften for 3 to 5 min.

5. For the sauce, ½ tsp oregano and ½ tsp garlic powder into the pan with the meat sauce and simmer for 5 min

6. Combine ricotta, ½ cup mozzarella, and ⅓ cup parmesan in a medium bowl.

7. Add a slight salt and pepper to taste and add the remaining oregano and garlic powder to the cheese mixture and fold until everything is well combined.

8. Turn off the heat and spread the meat over the pan until a uniform layer is left.

9. Place the Tbsp the cheese mixture around the pan, push them a little with your spoon at the bottom of the pan.

10. Sprinkle the top with the rest of the mozzarella and parmesan.

11. Bake for 20 min until boiling, and the top begins to brown.

12. Garnish with chopped parsley, if desired. Serve hot.

Steak and Pepper Salad

Servings: 5

Preparation Time: 15 minutes

Per Serving: 276 Calories; 15.3g Fat; 4.4g Carbs; 29g Protein; 1.1g Fiber

Ingredients:

- 1 ½ pounds beef sirloin steaks, sliced into bite-sized strips
- 2 bell peppers, sliced
- 2 tablespoons soy sauce
- 1 ½ tablespoons fresh lemon juice
- 2 tomatoes, sliced

Procedure:

1. Brush the sides and bottom of your wok with a nonstick cooking spray.
2. Then, stir fry the beef for 6 to 7 minutes, shaking the wok.

3. Add in peppers and continue to cook an additional 2 minutes or until the peppers are crisp-tender.

4. Place the cooked beef and pepper in a serving bowl.

5. Toss with the soy sauce, lemon juice, and tomatoes. Serve at and enjoy!

Classic Family Cheeseburger

Servings: 3

Preparation Time: 15 minutes

Per Serving: 533 Calories; 35.1g Fat; 4.8g Carbs; 46g Protein; 0.8g Fiber

Ingredients:

- 1 pound ground beef
- 3 slices Colby cheese
- 1 tablespoon olive oil
- 1 white onion, sliced
- 1 teaspoon burger seasoning mix

Procedure:

1. With oiled hands, mix the ground beef with the burger seasoning mix; season with salt and black pepper to taste.
2. Roll the mixture into 3 equal patties.
3. Heat the olive oil in a grill pan over medium-high heat.

4. Then, grill your burgers for 5 to 6 minutes, flipping them over with a a wide spatula.

5. Top with cheese and cook for 5 minutes more or until cheese has melted.

6. Serve with onions and enjoy!

Crockpot Porkloin

Servings: 8

Preparation Time: 8 10 minutes

Per Serving: Cal 561 Carbs 28g Protein 56g Fat 23g
Saturated Fat 11g

Ingredients:

- 3 ½ to 4-lb tenderloin
- ½ tsp garlic powder
- ¼ tsp ground ginger
- A pinch of dried thyme
- Salt and freshly ground black pepper
- 1 Tbsp cooking oil
- 2 cups chicken broth
- 2 Tbsp fresh lemon juice
- 1 Tbsp soy sauce
- 3 Tbsp cornstarch

Procedure:

1. Pour over the pork with the sauce.
2. Close the cooker gradually.
3. Cook 4 to 5 hours on low.

4. Pork Shoulder-Cook for 10 hours on low.

5. Remove pork from a serving plate and cover with foil loosely (10-20 min rest).

6. Pour all the juices into a large saucepan in a slow cooker. Add the mixture of cornflour steam, blend.

Thickened sauce:

7. Simmer for 5 min at medium-high or until it reduces to a consistency of syrup.

Roast Beef a la Cacerola

Servings: 5

Preparation Time: 40 minutes

Per Serving: 585 Calories; 40.1g Fat; 6.2g Carbs; 48g Protein; 1.1g Fiber

Ingredients:

- 5 ounces Chorizo sausage, chopped
- 2 eggs, whisked
- 2 pounds ground chuck
- 8 ounces Manchego cheese, grated
- 2 vine-ripe tomatoes, pureed

Procedure:

1. Melt 2 tablespoon of butter in a frying pan over a medium-high heat.
2. Brown Chorizo sausage and ground chuck for about 5 minutes until no longer pink.

3. Sprinkle with steak seasoning blend; add in tomatoes and stir to combine.

4. Continue to cook for 7 to 8 minutes over medium-low heat. Transfer the mixture into a buttered baking dish.

5. Top with Manchego cheese and bake for about 17 to 20 minutes or until hot and bubbly on the top. Enjoy!

Basil Lamb Shoulder with Pine Nuts

Servings: 4

Preparation Time: 1 hour

Per Serving: calories: 391 | fat: 33g | protein: 21g | carbs: 3g | net carbs: 2g | fiber: 1g

Ingredients:

- 1 pound (454 g) rolled lamb shoulder, boneless
- 1½ cups basil leaves, chopped
- 5 tablespoons pine nuts, chopped
- ½ cup green olives, pitted and chopped
- 3 cloves garlic, minced
- Salt and black pepper, to taste

Procedure:

1. Preheat the oven to 450°F.
2. In a bowl, combine the basil, pine nuts, olives, and garlic.
3. Season with salt and pepper.

4. Untie the lamb flat onto a chopping board, spread the basil mixture all over, and rub the spices onto the meat.

5. Roll the lamb over the spice mixture and tie it together using 3 to 4 strings of butcher's twine.

6. Place the lamb onto a baking dish and cook in the oven for 10 minutes.

7. Reduce the heat to 350°F and continue cooking for 40 minutes.

8. When ready, transfer the meat to a cleaned chopping board; let it rest for 10 minutes before slicing.

9. Serve with roasted root vegetables.

Crockpot Chili Verde

Servings: 12

Preparation Time: 30 minutes

Per Serving: Macros: 265 Cal; 12.4 g fat; 12.1 g Carbs; 22.5 g protein; 64 mg

Ingredients:

- 3 Tbsp olive oil
- ½ cup chopped onion
- 2 finely chopped garlic cloves
- 3 lbs boneless pork shoulder, diced
- 2 cans (7 oz) green sauce
- 1 can (4 g) cut jalapeno peppers
- 1 can (14.5 g) diced tomatoes

Procedure:

1. Heat the oil in a Dutch oven over medium heat.
2. Saute the onion and garlic.
3. Add the pork and cook until the outside is browned.

4. Add the green salsa, jalapeno peppers, and tomatoes in a slow cooker, and move the meat, onions, and garlic.

5. Cook for 3 hours on high.

6. Reduce setting to low and cook 4 to 5 more hours.

Asian Style Beef Brisket

Servings: 3

Preparation Time: 15 minutes

Per Serving: 277 Calories; 21.5g Fat; 2.7g Carbs; 17.4g Protein; 0.8g Fiber

Ingredients:

- 3/4 pound beef brisket, cut into small pieces
- 2 cups button mushrooms, sliced
- 3 scallions, sliced
- 1 celery, cut into matchsticks
- 1 teaspoon Five-spice powder

Procedure:

1. Heat 1 tablespoon of peanut oil in a medium-sized sauce pan over a medium-high heat.
2. Next, cook the beef brisket for 5 to 6 minutes, shaking the pan frequently.

3. Add a splash of Shaoxing wine (about 4 tablespoons) and deglaze the pan.

4. Stir in the mushrooms, scallions, and celery and continue to cook for 3 to 5 minutes more until they have softened.

5. Season with Five-spice powder. Enjoy!

Grilled Lamb Kebabs

Servings: 4

Preparation Time: 15 minutes

Per Serving: calories: 246 | fat: 15g | protein: 25g | carbs: 3g | net carbs: 2g | fiber: 1g

Ingredients:

- 1 pound (454 g) ground lamb
- ¼ teaspoon cinnamon
- 1 egg
- 1 onion, grated
- Salt and ground black pepper, to taste

Procedure:

1. Place all ingredients in a bowl.
2. Mix with your hands to combine well.
3. Divide the meat into 4 pieces.
4. Shape all meat portions around previously-soaked skewers.
5. Preheat grill to medium and grill the kebabs for about 5 minutes per side.

Dessert

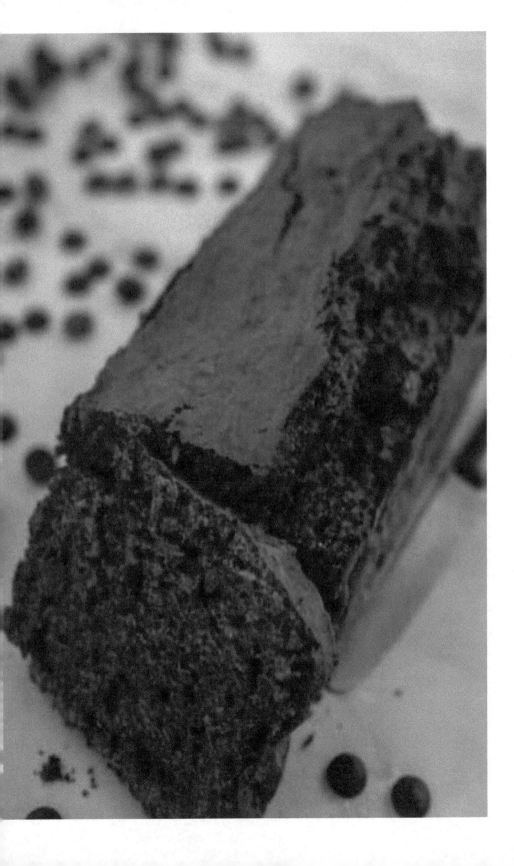

Chocolate Pound Cake

Servings: 12

Preparation Time: 30 minutes

Per Serving: 296 Calories; 27g Fat; 5.6g Carbs; 10.8g Protein; 2.7g Fiber

Ingredients:

- 1/3 cup cocoa powder, unsweetened
- 2 cups almond meal
- 1 cup coconut butter
- 2/3 cup full-fat milk, unsweetened
- 1 cup Swerve

Procedure:

1. Begin by preheating your oven to 365 degrees F.
2. Mix the almond meal, Swerve, and cocoa powder; add in 1 teaspoon of baking powder and stir again.
3. Add in the coconut butter and milk; add in butterscotch extract, if desired, and mix again until well combined.

4. Spoon the batter into a lightly buttered baking pan.
5. Bake in the preheated oven for about 20 minutes.
6. Place on a wire rack to cool and serve.

Tender Almond Pound Cake

Servings: 8

Preparation Time: 5-6 hours

Per Serving: calories: 281 | fat: 29g | protein: 5g | carbs: 1g | net carbs: 1g | fiber: 0g

Ingredients:

- 1 tablespoon coconut oil
- 2 cups almond flour
- 1 cup granulated erythritol
- ½ teaspoon cream of tartar
- Pinch salt
- 1 cup butter, melted
- 5 eggs
- 2 teaspoons pure vanilla extract

Procedure:

1. Lightly grease an 8-by-4-inch loaf pan with the coconut oil.
2. In a large bowl, stir together the almond flour, erythritol, cream of tartar, and salt, until well mixed.

3. In a small bowl, whisk together the butter, eggs, and vanilla.

4. Add the wet ingredients to the dry ingredients and stir to combine.

5. Transfer the batter to the loaf pan.

6. Place the loaf pan in the insert of the slow cooker.

7. Cover and cook until a toothpick inserted in the center comes out clean, about 5 to 6 hours on low.

8. Serve warm.

Pecan and Chocolate Cake

Servings: 9

Preparation Time: 25 minutes

Per Serving: 1.8 g net Carbs 2.6 g protein 7.1 g fat 3.4 g fiber 82.8 Cal

Ingredients:

- 29 g of protein powdered milk chocolate
- 1 Tbsp coconut flour
- A pinch of salt
- 2 Tbsp canned pumpkin
- 1 Tbsp maple syrup (sugar-free)
- 1 Tbsp coconut oil
- 1 tsp vanilla extract
- ¼ cup chopped nuts
- 6 Tbsp Lily's Sugar-Free Chocolate Chips
- 1 tsp coconut oil

Procedure:

1. In a small bowl, beat the protein powder, coconut flour, and salt.

2. Add the pumpkin puree, pancake syrup, coconut oil, and vanilla.

3. Mix with a fork until it begins to crumble, then mix the finely chopped nuts.

4. Divide it into 9 balls, it's easier to do by wrapping it in a Tbsp.

5. If the mixture crumbles too much and doesn't stick, add more pumpkin and a tsp at a time.

6. Roll into solid balls and place them in an airtight container in the freezer for 30 min

7. Heat the chocolate and coconut oil at 30-second intervals until it melts in a microwave-safe glass container (or heat it very carefully in a small box that fits into another container filled with ½ inch of water).

8. Stir until completely melted. Place a piece of parchment paper on a drawer, set aside.

9. Remove the balls from the freezer and immerse the nuts with 2 forks in the chocolate and place them in the pan.

10. If they are all covered, put them in the refrigerator for 30 min to cure them.

11. After hardening, keep the balls for up to a week in an airtight container in the fridge.

Basic Keto Brownies

Servings: 10

Preparation Time: 1 hour

Per Serving: 205 Calories; 19.5g Fat; 5.4g Carbs; 4.7g Protein; 3.2g Fiber

Ingredients:

- 1/2 cup coconut oil
- 3 ounces baking chocolate, unsweetened
- 5 tablespoons coconut flour
- 1/2 cup cocoa powder, unsweetened
- 4 eggs

Procedure:

1. Start by preheating your oven to 330 degrees F.
2. Thoroughly combine the coconut flour and cocoa powder; add in 1/2 teaspoon of baking powder.
3. Whisk the eggs with a keto sweetener, of choice; add in the melted coconut oil and chocolate.

4. Gradually stir the dry ingredients into the egg mixture, whisking constantly.

5. Scrape the batter into a buttered baking pan.

6. Bake in the preheated oven for 45 to 50 minutes or until a tester inserted into the middle of your brownie comes out dry. Enjoy!

Old Fashioned Gingerbread Cake

Servings: 8

Preparation Time: 3 hours

Per Serving: calories: 259 | fat: 23g | protein: 7g | carbs: 6g | net carbs: 3g | fiber: 3g

Ingredients:

- 1 tablespoon coconut oil
- 2 cups almond flour
- ¾ cup granulated erythritol
- 2 tablespoons coconut flour
- 2 tablespoons ground ginger
- 2 teaspoons baking powder
- 2 teaspoons ground cinnamon
- ½ teaspoon ground nutmeg
- ¼ teaspoon ground cloves
- Pinch salt
- ¾ cup heavy (whipping) cream
- ½ cup butter, melted
- 4 eggs
- 1 teaspoon pure vanilla extract

Procedure:

1. Lightly grease the insert of the slow cooker with coconut oil.
2. In a large bowl, stir together the almond flour, erythritol, coconut flour, ginger, baking powder, cinnamon, nutmeg, cloves, and salt.
3. In a medium bowl, whisk together the heavy cream, butter, eggs, and vanilla.
4. Add the wet ingredients to the dry ingredients and stir to combine.
5. Spoon the batter into the insert.
6. Cover and cook on low for 3 hours, or until a toothpick inserted in the center comes out clean.
7. Serve warm.

Haystack with Peanut Butter and Chocolate

Servings: 4

Preparation Time: 10 minutes

Per Serving: 1.1 g net Carbs 1.2 g protein 6.7 g fat 0.9 g fiber 74.9 Cal

Ingredients:

- ¼ cup heavy cream
- 2 Tbsp unsalted butter bar
- 3 Tbsp cocoa powder (sugar-free)
- 2 Tbsp xylitol
- 1/16 pinch of Stevia
- 1/16 tsp salt
- ¼ cup natural creamy peanut butter
- 2/3 cup coconut, grated, sugar-free

Procedure:

1. Combine cream, melted butter, cocoa powder, crystal sugar substitutes, and salt in a saucepan over medium heat.
2. Bring to a boil then remove from heat.

3. Add peanut butter and stir until it is absorbed.

4. Roast the coconut flakes in a saucepan at 350° For 5 min.

5. Once it is roasted, add the chocolate mixture until it is covered.

6. Place Tbsp on waxed paper or a silicone mat on a tray to form 18 mounds.

7. Let cool and harden or put in the fridge to dry quickly.

Avocado Chocolate Pudding

Servings: 2

Preparation Time: 5 minutes + chilling time

Per Serving: 163 Calories; 14.6g Fat; 9.8g Carbs; 4.7g Protein; 5.9g Fiber

Ingredients:

- 1/2 ripe avocado, pitted and peeled
- 2 ounces cream cheese
- 4 tablespoons unsweetened cocoa powder
- 4 tablespoons almond milk
- 1/4 cup swerve sweetener

Procedure:

1. Blend all of the above ingredients until well combined.
2. Serve in dessert bowls and enjoy!

Chocolate Brownie Cake

Servings: 12

Preparation Time: 3 hour 10 minutes

Per Serving: calories: 185 | fat: 16g | protein: 5g | carbs: 7g | net carbs: 6g | fiber: 1g

Ingredients:

- ½ cup plus 1 tablespoon unsalted butter, melted, divided
- 1½ cups almond flour
- ¾ cup cocoa powder
- ¾ cup granulated erythritol
- 1 teaspoon baking powder
- ¼ teaspoon fine salt
- 1 cup heavy (whipping) cream
- 3 eggs, beaten
- 2 teaspoons pure vanilla extract
- 1 cup whipped cream

Procedure:

1. Generously grease the insert of the slow cooker with 1 tablespoon of the melted butter.

2. In a large bowl, stir together the almond flour, cocoa powder, erythritol, baking powder, and salt.

3. In a medium bowl, whisk together the remaining ½ cup of the melted butter, heavy cream, eggs, and vanilla until well blended.

4. Whisk the wet ingredients into the dry ingredients and spoon the batter into the insert.

5. Cover and cook on low for 3 hours, and then remove the insert from the slow cooker and let the cake sit for 1 hour.

6. Serve warm with the whipped cream.

Chocolate Ice Cream

Servings: 4

Preparation Time: 20 minutes

Per Serving: 4.2 g net Carbs 3.2 g protein 24.6 g fat 1 g fiber 247.2 Cal

Ingredients:

- 2 cups heavy cream
- 4 large egg yolks
- 10 sachets of calorie-free sweeteners
- ¼ cup cocoa powder (sugar-free)
- 2 unsweetened chocolate syrup Tbsp
- 1 tsp vanilla extract

Procedure:

1. Heat the cream in a heavy saucepan over low heat.
2. Beat the egg yolks 1 by 1.
3. Cook over low heat, continually stirring until mixture covers the back of a spoon. Don't cook.

4. Keep away from heat.

5. Add the sugar substitute, cocoa powder, chocolate syrup, and vanilla extract.

6. Cool to room temperature. Freeze.

Peanut Butter Squares

Servings: 10

Preparation Time: 10 minutes

Per Serving: 122 Calories; 11.7g Fat; 4.9g Carbs; 1.5g Protein; 1.4g Fiber

Ingredients:

- 1 stick butter, room temperature
- 1/3 cup Swerve
- 1/2 cup unsweetened coconut flakes
- 1/3 cup unsweetened cocoa powder
- 1/3 cup peanut butter

Procedure:

1. Place the butter and peanut butter in your microwave for 30 seconds or until they have melted.
2. Stir in the other ingredients and mix again.
3. Pour the mixture into a foil-lined baking sheet.
4. Freeze for 1 hour or until firm enough to slice. Devour!

Coconut and Chocolate Fudge

Servings: 2

Preparation Time: 25 minutes

Per Serving: 405 Calories; 40g Fat; 8.8g Carbs; 6.3g
Protein; 5.3g Fiber

Ingredients:

- 1/4 cup coconut flour
- 1/3 cup coconut oil
- 2 ounces sugar-free dark chocolate, melted
- 2 tablespoons ground flax
- 1/3 cup xylitol

Procedure:

1. Thoroughly combine the ground flax, coconut flour,
   and xylitol in a bowl; add in 1/2 teaspoon of baking
   powder.
2. In a separate bowl, whisk the coconut oil and
   melted chocolate.

3. Stir the wet mixture into the dry mixture and mix until everything is well combined.

4. Scrape the batter in a foil-lined baking pan.

5. Bake in the preheated oven at 370 degrees F for about 20 minutes or until a toothpick comes out dry. Devour!

Chocolate and Nuts

Servings: 4

Preparation Time: 20 minutes

Per Serving: 0.9 g net Carbs 0.9 g protein 3.2 g fat 0.3 g fiber 35.7 Cal.

Ingredients:

- 2 Tbsp 100% stone whole grain puff pastry
- 2 Tbsp whole-grain soy flour
- A pinch of baking powder
- 3/4 cup sucralose sweetener (sugar substitute)
- 1 ½ oz sugar-free cooking squares
- 5 Tbsp heavy cream
- 2 Tbsp unsalted butter bar
- 2 large eggs
- 1 tsp vanilla extract
- ¼ cup chopped English walnuts

Procedure:

1. Preheat to 350° F. Roast the nuts lightly in an even layer on a baking sheet for 6 to 8 min.
2. Chill, chop the nuts, and save.

3. Set the oven to 375° F.

4. Cover 2 baking sheets with parchment paper or aluminum foil; put aside.

5. In a bowl, whisk 2 Tbsp whole wheat flour, 2 Tbsp soy flour, and baking powder; put aside.

6. In a large bowl of an electric mixer, beat eggs and sugar substitute over medium heat until soft and slightly thick.

7. Put the chocolate, cream, and butter in a microwave container; microwave over medium heat until butter melts and the chocolate becomes soft (no need to melt completely), 1½ to 2 min Let sit for 5 min.

8. Stir until smooth.

9. Gradually add the slightly hot chocolate mixture and vanilla extract to the egg mixture.

10. Reduce speed to low and add flour mixture only until everything is combined.

11. Cover and let cool 30 min

12. Place slightly rounded tsp, 1 inch apart, on the prepared sheet.

13. Sprinkle the top of the cookies with nuts, lightly press the dough.

14. Bake in the oven until cookies are ready but soft on top, 5½ to 6 min Cool the cookies on the baking sheet for 1 minute before moving them to the racks to cool them completely.

9 781803 259123